Survival Medicine & First Aid

• The Leading Prepper's Guide to Survive Medical Emergencies in Tough Survival Situations •

By Beau Griffin

Disclaimer

The author and publisher take no responsibility for any practical application of the information within this book, nor can they guarantee that the techniques described will be successful in the messy, unpredictable and stressful circumstances of an accident or injury. This book cannot replace medical training as a teaching guide to medicine and is not intended to do so. The reader is advised that we in no way recommend utilizing the advice in this book under ordinary circumstances when a true medical professional is or will soon be available. This book is intended only as a helping hand in the event that medical assistance is not, and will never be, available.

Table of Contents

Medicine After the Grid Goes Down

Imagine for a moment that an epidemic, a world war or a super event such as an eruption of the volcano under Yellowstone National Park has taken place. In the aftermath, few people have survived and all of those people are struggling to maintain their health and wellbeing on a day by day basis.

It's not hard to imagine – that, after all, is why you have picked up this book. You know all too well that the human race faces more potential disasters than we can count, ranging in severity from a localized incident such as an earthquake to a species destroying apocalypse. Many of us in fact believe that a world changing disaster is a case of "which one?" rather than "if".

In that brave new world, what's the one skill that will be most mourned? It's not farming or husbandry, because those can be re-learned with a little trial and error. It's not building or mending, because those too are so ingrained in the minds of most preppers that they will be widespread even among the few still living. It's not even reading or writing, because the majority of us can already do these things and can pass that knowledge down to the next generation.

The skill that we will bemoan the lack of most often in the aftermath of a huge disaster is, in fact, the ability to administer medicine and first aid. It's not a logical talent that we can simply figure out on the fly, it's not something that is understood by a large amount of the population and it quite literally means the difference between life and death. A doctor in the apocalypse will be worth their weight in gold to the survivors around them.

Unfortunately, there is no guarantee that you will be lucky enough to find a doctor in such a situation. In this book, we will be looking to fill that gap. Unless you or a family member is a doctor already or you have the good fortune to find yourself stranded with your local GP, medical care is something that you will definitely and desperately need in a world gone wild, one that is full of dangers and potential accidents.

Disaster medicine is not just a skill that counts in an apocalypse, either. In the scenario we just considered, there could be an extreme gap of time between the disaster taking place and the world going back to normal. But even in the case of a smaller disaster, two things remain true:

1 – You will be stranded for at least a period of time without access to medical facilities.

2 – You will be faced with higher levels of danger than you would during an ordinary day, leading to a greater potential for injuries and illness.

The difference between a small disaster and a long lasting apocalypse is that, in the latter, you will not have the choice to hand your patient over to a professional to finish the job. You, and only you, will be able to administer the aid that will hopefully help that person return to full health or, at the very least, give them the best possible chance of survival.

For this reason, we will cover both the basics of first aid and care for common everyday maladies in the pages of this guide. By the time you complete your studies of it, you will feel more confident in your ability to respond to an accident or an illness when there is no ambulance on call to do it for you.

Keep this book safe. For a medical professional, practice comes easy. For you, as you continue your normal life and its normal activities, it will be much harder to tend to your skills.

If you have built – or are planning to build – a shelter for your loved ones in the case of a wide scale disaster, make sure this book is stored within its library. It will serve as your bible, reminding you of the life saving techniques you may need.

If you are planning an excursion, a vacation or just an extended trip, bring this book with you. Again, you may find yourself grateful for the reminder if your plane goes down, an earthquake hits the city or a chemical spillage causes havoc.

Disasters happen every day. Hurricanes, tsunamis, avalanches and blizzards – take a look at the recent news and see how many you can pick out that would have left the people around them dearly in need of medical attention. Note that, for most of these incidents, the emergency services were stretched to breaking point and would have welcomed a helping hand from a knowledgeable bystander – if the emergency services had been able to respond in time at all.

The likelihood of a disaster happening near you is just high enough to make medicine an essential skill to know. By arming yourself with the knowledge in this book, you will be preparing yourself to fill that terrifying potential gap in human knowledge in the aftermath of a collapse. You will be the survivor who is worth their weight in gold, because you have the aptitude to administer the aid that is so sorely needed.

We cannot cover every single medical possibility and we cannot replace years of study as a medical student, but we can prepare you for the most likely injuries and illnesses you will face in either a small scale disaster or the collapse of society altogether. This book will specifically cover the problems that are most likely in the aftermath and the solutions that are most likely to be available to you. It won't make you a doctor – but it will make you a lifesaver.

Maintaining Your Health

As someone who is interested in making themselves ready to face the worst case scenario, you already know the value of preparation. You know that your chances of survival increase exponentially if you have provided options for water, food and shelter for yourself.

Ensuring that you – and every other member of your post collapse party – are healthy and fighting fit is very much in the same category of preparation. A healthy person is better able to fight off infection, heal from a fracture and avoid accidents.

The first piece of advice I will share with you is to become very conscious of your own body. Your health is always your greatest gift and will be even more so in the event of a disaster.

This advice applies to both you and every other member of your party – if you are aiming to shelter after a disaster with your spouse, kids, other family members and even friends, you will need to stress the importance of these things to them, too. Healthy patients are easier to treat, so think of this as preparing your patient ahead of time.

- Ascertain the correct weight and body fat ratio for your height, body type and age. Strive to reach this goal and pay attention to what you need to do to achieve it. This will bring you in tune with your body at its peak, telling you how many calories you must consume to maintain your health, the speed and efficiency of your metabolism and the level of exercise your particular body needs to stay at the same weight level. It will also bring you to optimum health and fitness levels, which will serve you well in a world of practical tasks and potential long journeys.

- Increase your levels of exercise. Most of us live a sedentary lifestyle – the same will not be true after a complete collapse. You will be called upon to fetch, carry, build, travel, climb and much more. Vary your exercise so that you are improving your strength, endurance and the flexibility of your body. Again, a body in excellent condition is more able to defend itself against disease and contamination and will heal more quickly after an accident.

- Review your diet and cut out as much junk and processed food as possible. Your diet after a disaster will eventually become dependent on the foods you can grow, gather and hunt – there will not be a fast food restaurant on every corner. If we're honest with ourselves, this is a good thing: fresh, whole foods leave our bodies in better condition than the junk meal alternative. Learn to pack your meals with the nutrients that keep your organs, skin, muscles and tissues strong and healthy. Be an expert on the foods that contain such minerals as iron and calcium in large quantities. Become a connoisseur of the healthful diet and watch your body respond positively to the change, once again improving your overall health and increasing your chances of staying healthy after a collapse.

- Schedule a yearly health panel with your doctor and make sure to review it thoroughly with them. Watch for the early signs of problems such as cancer, liver problems, high cholesterol, diabetes, high or low blood pressure and heart disease and ensure that you tackle them head on to prevent them from becoming an issue. It's tough to get your hands on insulin after a disaster – much better to have spotted the danger early and prevented it from fully taking form.

- In the case of unavoidable health issues (and it's important we acknowledge that we cannot always stave off the inevitable), be sure to develop as much knowledge as possible. Know what medications are necessary and how to administer them; know whether there are alternatives that can be found in a scenario that includes a lack of hospitals and medical care. You should also know what situations and activities could aggravate a condition, which will better help you to prevent that from happening. For example, low oxygen environments such as high altitudes can affect many ongoing conditions, such as heart problems and lung disease. Medicine in a post collapse world is a very personal journey – it's your job right now to identify the types of illness and injury you are likely to face and be prepared to handle them.

- Immunize yourself against as many of the most common forms of disease as possible, such as malaria. Make sure to keep these immunizations up to date. Even if the disaster you find yourself faced with does not begin with an epidemic, illness spreads alarmingly quickly when the grid goes down. It can be carried in the water, between survivors – even in the air. The more illnesses you develop an immunity to now, the fewer you will have to tackle after the collapse.

First Aid Vs. Survival Medicine

As we said at the beginning of this book, there is a difference between administering first aid to an injured person after an earthquake while you wait for the first responders to arrive and caring for a person from the moment they become sick or injured right through until they make a full recovery.

It's relatively easy to find first aid courses that are open to the general public. In the UK, for example, St. John's Ambulance provides voluntary first aid care at events and is always looking for volunteers. In the U.S., most volunteer ambulance departments are constantly seeking new recruits. In many countries, the Red Cross teaches first aid, often with a specific focus on disasters.

If you wish to bolster your knowledge of first aid and give yourself some practical experience, seeking out such a course is a great idea. Be aware, however, that there are few courses being taught out there that don't make one very important assumption: that you, as the first aid giver, will eventually be able to hand your patient over to someone with greater experience and more available equipment.

Therein lies the difference between first aid and survival medicine. It's important to grasp this difference fully, because it's also one of the first things you will need to ascertain if you are called on to use your medicinal skills.

First Aid

First aid is the immediate response to an injury or sudden illness. It tackles any danger of the patient dying before help can properly be administered and aims to ensure the patient is given the best possible chance to not only survive, but to survive intact.

First aid is an essential skill because it will always be your immediate response to a serious medical problem. You will, after all, always need to diagnose the problem and remove any immediate danger that the issue could cause further damage and even death.

Should you find yourself in the path of an avalanche, faced with a climbing or hiking accident in the wilderness or dealing with survivors after an earthquake, your first aid skills will follow the strategy known to every first responder in the world: stabilize the patient ready for transportation. Basically, you are preparing the injured person to be taken to a medical facility for more in depth treatment.

Outback Medicine

There is an interim scenario between first aid and survival medicine. Not every disaster occurs within a city or civilized region. Let's say, for example, that you are involved in a plane crash and asked to provide aid for a fellow survivor, knowing that help could take hours, days or even weeks to arrive.

Should you find yourself stranded far from civilization, you will become that patient's best and perhaps only chance for survival. You will still need to administer first aid – diagnosing and providing immediate treatment for the problem – but you will also need to factor in the follow-up care that will keep the person stable until help does arrive.

Survival Medicine

The third and final scenario assumes that help is not coming at all. This is a safe assumption in the case of a large scale disaster that cuts you off from civilization or leaves you as one of very few survivors.

In this scenario, you are not just needed at the site of the initial injury. You will not only need to stabilize the injury and ensure the patient is given the best possible chances of a full recovery. After a collapse, you *are* that patient's best chance of a full recovery and you will need to continue your care until the injury or illness is completely cured or controlled.

This will also apply to conditions that are already present or that manifest after the disaster. You will need to be able to tackle chronic conditions such as arthritis, thyroid problems and heart disease as well as illnesses such as the flu and chicken pox.

As will no doubt have become clear, survival medicine is an all-encompassing skill with a different approach to basic first aid. For this reason, we will be covering both scenarios in this book to prepare you as fully as possible for what may come.

Your First Aid Strategy

For any first responder to an illness, accident or injury, there is a basic order of duties that must always be followed. As the primary caregiver in a situation, whether it's a car crash or a full collapse of civilization, it will be your job to provide that instant response and to do it in such a way that both you and your patient emerge in good condition.

Because your safety and the safety of your patient are important and your aim is to make sure the person you are treating survives, this set of principles must become your mantra. Any and every time you are faced with a need to employ your skills, whether you are administering first aid until help arrives or you will be caring for the patient in the long term, these are the steps you must follow.

- Assess the situation. Cast a discerning eye over the scene you are faced with, looking for any dangers and hazards to either yourself or your patient. Ensure, for example, that you will not be hit by debris or injured yourself while trying to reach your patient.

- Remove immediate dangers. Before you begin administering treatment, do everything in your power to prevent the situation from becoming worse. Your safety is as important as the patient's – if you, too, are injured, their chances of survival are lost. Extinguish fires, remove loose debris and move your patient to a safer location if you cannot secure the scene itself.

- Protect yourself from contamination. As you do not yet know with full confidence what you are dealing with, make sure to protect yourself before you administer aid. A face mask, gloves and an apron are all important medical tools, not only to prevent contaminated fluids from contact with you, but also to protect your patient from contamination from your own body.

- Assess for threats to life. In that first instant, you do not need to know the full extent of your patient's injuries. What you need to know first is whether any aspect of this situation will threaten the patient's life. It's no use diagnosing a compound fracture, for example, if your patient bleeds out in the meantime from a severed artery. You will need to check:

Airway – is there anything blocking the person's mouth or throat and preventing them from inhaling oxygen?

Breathing – is the patient breathing normally?

Circulation – is the patient's heart still beating normally? Is there any bleeding severe enough to cause a threat to life?

Extreme injury – has the patient suffered a neck or head injury that must be stabilized to ensure survival?

Exposure – is the patient exposed to any external or environmental threat that could threaten their life?

- Treat life threatening issues. Deal with any life threatening issues you have identified immediately, before continuing with your diagnosis and first aid. Ensure the patient is stabilized before you begin a deeper examination.

- Perform a thorough investigation. Your patient may or may not be able to communicate their injuries to you. If they are conscious, ask them to tell you what happened and where they hurt. This will provide you with at least some information to help your diagnosis but be aware that your patient may not be aware of every injury affecting them. Not all issues cause pain and some can cause numbness or paralysis. Examine the body thoroughly to be sure you are aware of less obvious issues and are able to provide initial treatment for them.

- Administer aid. Perform first aid on any wounds, breakages and other problems, such as shock and hypothermia. Your aim here is to stabilize the patient to give them the best chance possible of a recovery. Except in extreme conditions, the patient's long term care will take place in a secondary location.

- Plan for evacuation. If help is on the way, your contribution may not reach this stage. If it is not, consider where and how you will transport the patient to a safe location and how you will prevent any part of their injuries from worsening in the process.

- Transport the patient. Ensure that your patient is stable and secure before moving them. Particularly if there is a neck or back injury, moving the person can cause severe damage.

You may need to consider creating a shelter where you are so that you can treat the patient in place. If you feel that they are stable enough to be moved, make sure you have secured any broken limbs and that any bandages or wound coverings will stay in place.

The Principles of First Response

All the while that you are following the guidelines we covered in the last chapter to successfully treat a patient at the scene of an accident or injury, there is a set of principles that any first aider should aim to follow. These principles strive to improve your chances of success – and to leave your patient in the best condition you can leave them in.

- Stay calm. Though not always an easy guideline to follow, this is imperative. You will make better decisions, notice more details and be more productive in a calm state of mind – when we hurry, we make considerably more mistakes. Not to mention the effect that your reaction will have on the patient – the last thing you want is an injured person panicking, attempting to move and in the process worsening their injuries and negatively affecting their own heart rate.

- Involve the patient. As we briefly mentioned earlier, your patient knows better than you do exactly what happened to them, so their help can be invaluable. They can also tell you of hidden issues that could affect your treatment;

for instance, perhaps they have a blood clotting disease that will increase the time it takes for a wound healing over on its own. Perhaps they feel nauseated or their head is throbbing – these are symptoms you cannot see, but that can help you reach an accurate diagnosis. Involving the patient has the secondary outcome of keeping them calm and quelling their fears. It is only respectful, after all, to ask for permission before you begin treatment and to keep them appraised of your progress. No matter how good your intentions, remember that this is not your body and you do not have an automatic right to touch it.

- Seek information. Whether or not your patient can communicate with you, there are still clues to their condition you can look for. Always assess the scene with an eye to causality: what exactly led to these injuries, and why? In many cases, this can lead to a better diagnosis or even allow you to spot more subtle injuries. It's also a good idea to check for medical cards or bracelets that might alert you to pre-existing conditions.

- Assume the worst. Pessimism is not often thought of as a positive trait, but it's certainly useful in a first aid situation. You may not be able to tell yet whether your patient is suffering from hidden injuries or a broken neck or back, so it's always a good idea to assume that these problems are present. Better to go the extra mile to move a patient onto a stretcher than to discover too late, as you help them stand, that a neck injury was present all along.

- Enlist help. Speed can be of the essence in a crisis, both to ensure the patient's survival and to complete your treatment and move the patient to a safer location as quickly as possible. Bystanders and your own companions may not be medically trained, but they can still assist you in many of the tasks you will be called on to perform. In particular, it's seldom a good idea to try to move a patient on your own unless you have no choice.

- Take charge. With that said, too many cooks have a habit of spoiling the broth. If you are enlisting help, be clear when you establish yourself as the medical authority in this situation. Announce that you are taking charge as a first responder and have the situation under control, using an authoritative tone. Request assistance and explain clearly what you need and why. Of course, it's perfectly fine to relinquish your authority if you discover that there is a qualified medical professional within the group – deferring to greater knowledge and experience is never a bad idea.

- Consider all dangers. Accidents rarely happen in safe locations. Crashes, falls, even the disaster itself – all of these things have the potential to harm you and anyone else at the scene. Do not put yourself or anyone else in harm's way without good reason. Throwing yourself in a churning river and being swept away to your own death will not save the victim and it is your responsibility and duty to make sure you do not endanger any bystanders or helpers by asking them to take on the danger for you. While treating the patient, continue to be alert for dangers and make sure your priority is to move everyone to a safer location.

- **Think hard before you move your patient.** Only if a patient is in danger where they are or is recovered enough to be moved should you consider any form of travel. Walking or even the process of being carried can exacerbate problems to the point that you will no longer be able to treat them. Whether or not to move your patient will be perhaps the most difficult choice you have to make. Gather all your information and complete a thorough diagnosis before you even consider it.

First Aid and Medical Supplies

As the person responsible for medicine and first aid within your group, you will also be responsible for ensuring that your shelter or kit bag is equipped for administering care. You are going to need plenty of supplies within your grasp and enough of those supplies to last for the amount of time you will be unable to obtain help from a hospital.

In other words, if you are heading out on an excursion, you will need enough supplies to last for a few days, before help arrives. If you are stocking a shelter that will become a permanent residence after a collapse, you will need to be able to provide aid for months, if not years.

For everyday maladies and small problems, you will need:

- Painkillers (and a child friendly version if you will have younger housemates)
- Aspirin for aches, pains and heart problems
- Benadryl for allergic reactions
- Adrenaline injectors
- Diarrhea medicine
- Cough and sore throat medicine
- Flu and severe cold remedies

- Antibiotics
- Women's menstrual products (if you or your female companions are willing, you can purchase washable versions instead of disposable)
- Diapers and baby care products
- A good quality skin lotion
- Stomach upset remedy
- Antacids
- Electrolyte replacement powder/ oral rehydration salts (for use after vomiting or diarrhea)
- Calamine lotion
- Burn spray or gel
- Moleskin
- Aloe vera gel for sunburn
- Silver sulfadiazine cream
- Potassium iodide tablets
- Celox combat gauze
- Soap and hand sanitizer
- Topical antifungal powder or ointment
- Steroid cream
- Antihistamines
- A supply of any medications you or a member of your party must take regularly, such as insulin or heart medication.

For the first aid treatment of wounds and other emergencies:

- Plenty of bandages (these will need to be changed regularly, so expect to go through plenty even for a single injury)
- Band Aids and dressings
- Butterfly bandages
- Hemostatic bandages to control severe blood loss
- Medical grade glue
- Antibiotic ointment
- Sterile gauze
- Sterile dressings
- Medical tape
- Disinfectant, such as rubbing alcohol, to clean wounds
- Towels
- Splints and wraps for all limbs in case of breakages or sprains
- Scalpels and a field knife
- A hemostat clamp
- Hemostatic products for serious bleeds e.g. blood stopper bandages, hemostatic gauze
- A nylon suture
- Eye pads
- A neck clamp

- A tourniquet
- A neck collar
- Oxygen tank
- An epinephrine auto injector for severe allergic reaction
- Asthma inhaler (bronchodilator)
- Corticosteroid tablets
- Anticoagulant (enoxaparin or heparin)
- Maintenance anticoagulant (dabigatran or rivaroxaban)
- Activated charcoal.

For general equipment within your medical room:

- A thermometer – preferably two, one oral and one rectal
- A stethoscope
- Latex or rubber gloves (if you opt for latex, be sure to check that none of your party is allergic to the material)
- A surgical mask for use during first aid and surgery
- Sterile gloves
- Scalpels and scalpel blades of various sizes
- A tourniquet
- Syringes and injection needles
- Sterilizing wipes to clean wounds
- An airway

- Tweezers
- Scissors
- A small flashlight, pen light or head lamp
- A blood pressure cuff
- Medical needle and thread for stitching wounds
- Safety pins
- Petroleum jelly
- Cotton balls
- A glucose meter
- A blood pressure cuff
- Bandages and dressings in every shape and size you are able to find
- Compression wraps
- A thermal blanket to treat hypothermia
- Cold and hot compresses for swelling
- Crutches and walking sticks to aid motion after a sprain, fracture or other injury
- A stretcher.

Though many of these items are easily found in pharmacies and even supermarkets, or can be ordered on the internet, you may find that you are unable to locate some of them. Do not worry: make it a priority after a disaster to locate a medical supply center. Find out now where the nearest one is to your shelter.

You can both shore up your supplies and fill any gaps by doing this, often getting your hands on antibiotics and other medicines that are not usually available to the layperson. Though it is never recommended to administer such treatments under normal circumstances without proper medical training, a disaster scenario calls for different behavior.

Immediate Signals and Vital Signs

Never assume that you are seeing the full extent of the damage when you first encounter a patient. He or she may complain of nothing more serious than a bruised knee, but that doesn't mean you are safe to assume that nothing else is wrong. After all, we've all heard the stories of internal bleeding that went unnoticed until it was too late and the broken ankle that was walked on for two days before anyone noticed.

A first responder should always aim to make an assessment of the patient's full body, from head down to toe. Assume the worst – a criminal might be innocent until proven guilty, but a first responder knows that an injury is guilty until proven innocent.

Your primary indicator of a patient's status will be their vital signs: heart beat, breathing and blood pressure. As you begin your assessment of the situation, these are the details you will want to focus on.

Vital signs, of course, vary according to the patient's age. In general, look for vital signs in these ranges:

- For a newborn baby, expect 30 to 50 breaths per minute, a pulse somewhere between 120 and 160 beats per minute and blood pressure of 60 to 80.

- For a baby aged six months to a year, expect 30 to 40 breaths per minute, a pulse somewhere between 110 and 140 beats per minute and blood pressure of 70 to 80.

- For a toddler aged two to four, expect 20 to 30 breaths per minute, a pulse somewhere between 100 and 110 beats per minute and blood pressure of 80 to 95.

- For a child aged five to eight years, expect 14 to 20 breaths per minute, a pulse somewhere between 90 and 100 beats per minute and blood pressure of 90 to 100.

- For a child aged eight to 12 years, expect 12 to 20 breaths per minute, a pulse somewhere between 80 and 100 beats per minute and blood pressure of 100 to 110.

- For a teenager aged 12 to 18 years, expect 12 to 20 breaths per minute, a pulse somewhere

between 60 and 90 beats per minute and blood
pressure of 100 to 120.

- For an adult, expect 12 to 18 breaths per
  minute, a pulse somewhere between 55 and 90
  beats per minute and blood pressure of 120.

Your initial examination of a patient needs to check
off all the likely indicators of a problem. As a general
rule, you can follow these steps to thoroughly
investigate the person's health and status:

- Check for breathing. If your patient is not
  awake, place your ear near the nose and mouth
  to see if you can hear breath moving in and
  out. Watch their chest at the same time. Count
  the breaths according to the person's vital
  signs. If the person is not breathing or is
  struggling to breathe, you will need to open
  the airway or breathe on their behalf. It is
  absolutely vital to steady the breathing first as
  your patient cannot go long without oxygen. If
  you hear noises such as a rattle in the
  breathing, there may be an obstruction in the
  throat that will need to be removed.

- Check the pulse. Use the tip of your middle
  and index fingers to check for a pulse on the

artery at the patient's wrist. If you cannot find one, check the inside of the upper arm (brachial artery), groin (femoral artery) or neck (carotid artery). If you are unable to find a pulse, you will need to administer chest compressions immediately.

- Look for bleeding. Breathing and heartbeat should always be checked first for an unconscious patient, but a conscious one clearly has these functions to at least a good enough degree to be capable of speech. When dealing with a conscious patient, begin a dialogue with them as soon as possible to reassure them of your intentions and gather input from them. Meanwhile, look for bleeding. Any site of bleeding can be harmful, but heavy bleeding can be deadly very quickly. Examine the patient from head to toe to identify any areas of heavy bleeding. These must be addressed as soon as possible.

- Perform a full body evaluation. Move clothing as much as you are able without unnecessarily exposing the patient. Look for obvious abnormalities anywhere on the body that could indicate fractures, wounds and other issues.

- Check the patient's mental status. If the patient is awake and speaking, you should ask questions such as name, profession, date and other facts to determine how lucid they are. Listen to the speech: if there is any abnormality, such as slurring, this could be a symptom of a problem such as hypothermia.

- Check the blood pressure. The average blood pressure of a person at rest is 140/90. Too low may indicate shock or that your patient is hemorrhaging.

- Feel the patient's neck. Gently check the vertebra and look for tenderness and muscles in spasm. Also check the Adam's apple for a sensation almost like crunching. If you suspect any possibility of a neck injury, immobilize the neck as quickly as possible. Sudden movement can exacerbate the problem and pain can cause a patient to twitch or try to move.

- Check the spine. To look for back injuries, run your fingers down the spine, pressing gently to check for tender areas. Ask the patient to move their limbs and tell you if they have lost feeling in any areas. You can also pinch fingers and toes to check that the patient still has sensation. Any loss of feeling may indicate a back injury that will require the patient to be immobilized as securely as possible – and kept in one position unless necessary.

- Check for head injuries. Press the scalp gently to look for any areas where the skull or skin is raised or depressed and look for any bleeding or abrasions. Shine a light into the patient's eyes to check that the pupils are of equal size and respond to the light by constricting. If the pupils are small, this could be a sign of a brain injury or an overdose, while uneven pupils can mean the eye itself is injured or can also indicate head injury. Meanwhile, check for breaks and other problems on the head, such as a broken nose, loose teeth or a swollen tongue.

- Look at the skin. Check for such indicators as sweat, an abnormal skin color, bruises, rashes, bites or burns. Feel the temperature to check for fever. Check for circulation by pressing down on a fingernail so that the skin goes white; if the circulation is normal, color will return within two seconds. Pinching the skin and seeing it remain loose may indicate dehydration. Check inside the eyelids for a pale color that can indicate there is internal bleeding or anemia.

- Check the patient's chest. Feel the chest for tender areas or deformities and observe it to check that it is expanding and contracting fully and evenly with each breath the patient takes.

- Inspect the abdomen. Again, check for any cuts and wounds and press to see if there is any tenderness.

- Check limbs and joints. Press each arm and leg as well as the chest, ribs and collarbone to look for tenderness and breaks.

- Take the patient's temperature. Abnormalities in a person's core temperature can be a strong indicator that all is not well with the patient's body. Too low may indicate a condition such as hypothermia, while too high may indicate hyperthermia or fever.

These steps will allow you to evaluate the patient and check for symptoms of specific problems – more on these later in the book. If the patient is well enough to move, ask them to come with you to shelter and observe them for hours or days, depending on the severity of the injuries, to check for any deterioration and administer follow up care.

Whether or not you need to keep the patient from moving, it's best to always assume that the situation will deteriorate with time. Make sure to repeat your examinations regularly to look for new signs and signals and check that the symptoms you have identified have not worsened or spread.

Also, you should continue to check the mental situation of the patient, to ensure that he or she remains lucid. Again, assume that the situation is likely to deteriorate with time. Try not to leave the patient alone unless absolutely necessary – if you must leave to fetch supplies or tend to a second victim, be sure to leave a volunteer to watch over them.

Dealing With Multiple Casualties

The best case scenario for an emergency responder who must work alone to help a patient is that you will only need to deal with the needs of one person. Unfortunately, especially in a survival situation, that won't always be the case.

That's where triage comes in: a time honored practice used by medical professionals when they are overwhelmed by the sheer numbers of injured or sick people they must help as quickly as possible.

In this scenario, follow these guidelines:

- Assess for safety. Earthquakes often have aftershocks. Damage to a building can mean delayed falling of debris. A disaster could cause a fire to spark. Never assume that you are safe to run in and begin helping your patients – and always assume that they will ultimately be better off if you are safe and whole. Many people have trouble with this concept – it can feel plain wrong to put your own safety above that of the injured. Remember that you are these people's sole hope for medical attention and putting yourself in danger is very much against their interests.

- **Assess the scene.** How many patients are you dealing with? What type of injuries are you seeing and how severe are they? Is there anyone else at the scene who might be able to help you? Is there an area nearby that you could use to gather the injured together?

- **Ask for help.** If you have any form of communication device, summon help as quickly as possible. If you need someone to bring medical supplies for you, specify what you will need. If there are uninjured people on scene, ask for their help and ascertain how much medical training they have, which will dictate how they can assist you. Make it clear that you are in command of this situation – unless there is a more experienced medical professional nearby.

- **Set up your treatment area.** Find the best possible place to bring patients together in one place after you have made sure they can safely be moved.

- Perform a primary evaluation. Your first examination of each patient needs to be quick but thorough. At this moment, your goal is to determine which patients need your help first and which can be left a little longer without too much danger to their life. Check for breathing and heartbeat, check that the circulation is adequate and check the patient's mental status. Check for extreme bleeding – this, and clearing any blockages to a patient's airway, is the only actual treatment you should perform at this moment. Place your patients in priority order – if you are able to tag them, as medical professionals do in a triage situation, this can help you quickly move between patients later. Even a simple mark on their forehead with a pen can make things quicker for you as time moves on.

* Red – Immediate help needed. This patient will not survive if aid is not administered immediately and is therefore your top priority.

* Yellow – This person will need your help within the next couple of hours as their wounds could threaten their life if left untreated any longer, but they can safely wait

47

for you to administer aid to your red tag patients.

* Green – This patient has no life threatening wounds and will require only minimal treatment once you have been able to administer to the more seriously injured.

* Black – The hardest tag to apply, this means that the patient is either already dead or is not likely to survive.

- Begin treatment. Start with your red tag patients and move as quickly as you can to treat the serious and life threatening injuries affecting them. Your goal in a triage situation is not to completely treat every single wound, but to quickly ensure that person will survive so that you can move on to helping the next. You will then come back to that patient later to complete your treatment. The more patients you have, the less time you have to work with. Ask your helpers to move your patients into the treatment area you identified earlier as soon as you are confident they can be moved without causing damage. If you do not have a stretcher available, insert two strong poles in the arms or legs of any strong piece of clothing to create a makeshift one. Show your helpers how to move the person onto the stretcher, by grasping the shoulders of their shirt or jacket, allowing their head to rest on the forearms and pulling gently without too much vertical movement or bending of the neck or spine. For less seriously injured patients, use a fireman's lift: place the arms under the patient's arms, put one foot firmly between their legs, grasp the right wrist with the left hand and place it over your right shoulder, place your right hand between the legs and around the right thigh and lift them with their torso over your back.

Life Saving Techniques

The first category of treatment we will look at deals with the injuries and issues that could threaten a person's life. As a first responder, these are likely the techniques you will use first and foremost with a seriously injured patient.

Clearing an Airway

If your patient has vomited or their mouth and throat is blocked, they will be unable to breathe and will quickly become unconscious and then die. If your patient is unable to speak, appears panicked, has blue tinged skin or you can hear rasping and whistling as they breathe, gently lift the jaw forwards and upwards without moving the neck in case of injury. If there is no chance of a neck injury, place one hand under the person's neck and the other on their forehead to gently tilt back the head, which will open the airway as much as possible.

Now, sweep two fingers in the patient's mouth to check for any objects obstructing the breath. If the person is choking on their own tongue, you will need to pull it forward and out of the mouth and, in extreme circumstances, you may need to use a safety pin through the tongue and cheek to keep it from falling back down over the throat.

If an object is lodged in the throat and cannot be grasped properly with your fingers without the danger of forcing it further down, use tweezers to remove it. If you cannot do this, sit the victim up and use your open palm to hit them on the back up to four times firmly to dislodge the item.

Heimlich Maneuver

If your victim is choking and you are unable to retrieve the object with tweezers or slapping the back, you can also attempt the Heimlich maneuver if necessary. From behind the patient, clasp your hands around the upper abdomen, just below the ribs. Squeeze suddenly and very firmly then release. Do this two or three times to elicit a cough and ejection of the object in the throat. If this does not work, follow by slapping three to four times on the back and then repeat the Heimlich maneuver.

If the patient cannot stand, sit astride their lower body and place your hands, one on top of the other, over the abdomen. Press down suddenly and firmly and then check the mouth to remove the object.

If you are the person choking, it is possible to perform a Heimlich maneuver on yourself. Find a sturdy surface the height of your abdomen and throw yourself against it to produce the same reaction as your hands would on a patient.

Mouth to Mouth Resuscitation

If your patient is not breathing, you will need to do this for them – a lack of oxygen to the brain for any more than a couple of minutes will cause irreversible brain damage. Tilt the head backwards to open the airway, check the mouth for obstructions and then pinch the nose closed with your fingers.

Cover the patient's mouth with your own (preferably while wearing a surgical mask for your own protection). Blow air into the person's mouth until their chest rises – a full breath, which should take around two seconds. Remove your mouth from theirs to allow them to exhale, then repeat.

Be sure not to force the air into the lungs too hard, particularly with small children and babies. Repeat this cycle until help arrives or the patient begins breathing on their own. If you are encountering any difficulty blowing air into the lungs, this generally means there is an obstruction you will need to remove.

In some circumstances, mouth to mouth resuscitation can cause the stomach to fill up with enough air that it becomes tense and hinders your efforts. If this occurs, turn the patient on their side and press on the abdomen. If this causes vomiting, clean out their mouth before continuing.

CPR

If the patient has no heartbeat, you can pump the heart on their behalf. Kneel next to the patient's chest and place your hands, one on top of the other, over the center of the patient's breast bone. Interlock your fingers. The heel of your lower hand should be approximately the width of two fingers above the bottom edge of the patient's breast bone.

Line your shoulders up over your hands and keep your arms straight at the elbow. Keep your arms straight as you compress the breast bone around two inches and then release. You should be aiming for a speed that will provide around 100 compressions in one minute. Regularly check for a pulse and breathing; if none is found, continue your efforts.

For an infant, use one hand to hold the child's back and the other to perform compressions. Your compression depth should be shallower at around 1.5 inches.

Combining CPR and Mouth to Mouth

In many cases, you will find that a patient without a heartbeat also is not breathing. In this scenario, perform 30 chest compressions and then administer two breaths using the mouth to mouth technique.

Repeat this cycle until help arrives or the person begins breathing on their own. If you have a second helper, one person should administer the breath and the other administer the compressions to save switching time between the two techniques.

Treating Shock

Shock is a common reaction to a serious injury and is a condition you should keep a close eye out for as you treat that patient. If they do go into shock, it can be life threatening as the circulatory system is no longer providing sufficient oxygenated blood to the patient's body. This, in turn, leads to oxygen deprivation across the body.

Watch for changes to the patient's skin: it will likely become clammy and pale. The patient may sweat and exhibit shallow, fast breathing as well as feel weak, dizzy and nauseated. Watch for sighing and yawning as well as feelings of thirst.

Lay the patient down and raise their legs into an elevated position (unless they have a severe head injury or a spinal injury). Cover them with a warm blanket and continue to speak to them reassuringly. Administer oxygen at a rate of 10 liters every minute using a face mask.

Recovery Position

Once you are satisfied that the patient has no neck or back injuries and that your patient is breathing and has no other injuries that could prove life threatening, it's usually a good idea to move them into the recovery position. This position makes sure that their airway stays clear because any vomit or other fluids that congregate in the mouth and throat can escape thanks to simple gravity.

With the patient laying on their back, kneel beside them and place the arm closest to you at a right angle to their body, with the hand pointing up towards their head. Tuck the other hand beside their cheek on the same side and bend the knee furthest from you up and over so that it is across the leg that is closest to you. Roll the patient towards you by pulling the knee. If they are correctly positioned, their face should be supported by one hand and the knee and bottom arm will prevent them from rolling any further.

First Aid to Treat Serious Injuries

Serious injuries can be defined as the type of wound or injury that is either immediately a threat to the patient's life or could become a threat if left too long without care. These are the injuries that you, as a medical care giver, should watch for during that initial diagnosis after an accident or in the aftermath of a disaster.

The most serious injuries should always be treated first, obviously. These techniques can mean the difference between life and death and will stabilize the patient, allowing you to begin diagnosing additional problems or treating other injuries.

In some cases, these treatments are a first step only and you will need to revisit the wound later, once the patient has been moved to a safe place. Keep in mind that your goal is to save the patient's life, so these first aid techniques are intended to stabilize injuries and prevent them from worsening.

Protection of the Neck and Spine

A neck or spinal injury can be deadly or, at the very least, cause permanent paralysis. A first responder must be conscious at all times of the possibility that such an injury exists. If there is a chance that the spine or neck has been broken or injured, immediately immobilize the patient's head. Symptoms of this will include an inability to move the next or lower body, extreme pain or weakness and numbness and a loss of control of the bladder or bowels.

Apply a sturdy neck collar. In the absence of this piece of equipment, place two rolled towels on either side of the head and use a wide bandage across the forehead to secure it. Use another towel around the neck to keep it from moving.

If you need to align the head with the neck to secure it, be extremely careful with your movement and stop if you feel the slightest resistance. Rotate the head with both hands, starting by moving it so that the neck is not bent sideways without attempting to rotate the head. If your patient is conscious, ask them to alert you to any pain or change in their condition as you do this. Be extremely careful not to flex the patient's neck forward or backward as you move it.

If the victim must be moved, either to a safer location or to allow them to vomit, grasp the shoulders while holding the head between your forcarms as you do so. This will keep the head stabilized. You can use this method to move the patient onto a back board or stretcher, allowing them to be transported safely without further movement of the spine.

If your patient appears to have a spinal injury and you cannot slide a backboard underneath them, use the "logroll" technique. Have one person secure the head and neck, making sure to keep both in a fixed position at all times. To do this, the second person should extend one arm above the patient's head, which the first person should take hold of and use to support one side of the head and neck, while aligning their other forearm along the other side of the head and grasping the shoulder.

The patient's second arm should be placed along their body. Both helpers should then turn the patient gently and carefully onto their side (with the arm extended along the body moving upwards). The backboard or stretcher can be place on the ground before gently and carefully rolling the patient back onto it.

Severe Blood Loss

Unsurprisingly, your main priority if your patient is losing blood heavily is to stem the flow of that blood loss as quickly as you can. First, check that there is nothing inside the wound – it's common for shrapnel from whatever punctured the skin to become embedded. Be very careful before removing an embedded item from the wound as doing so can "unplug" the wound. If the item is plugging an artery, you could considerably worsen the bleeding.

Instead, you will be better served by securing the bleeding now and removing the foreign object later, when you are able to see it more clearly and the patient is in a safe place and has been treated for any other injuries. To do this, press firmly on either side of the shrapnel and pad around it before bandaging the wound.

If the wound is clear, use a dressing to press down firmly until the bleeding stops, applying pressure to the wound. Once the bleeding slows, use a new dressing to firmly and tightly bandage the wound. If the wound continues to bleed or begins to bleed anew, do not remove the dressing. Apply pressure to stop the bleeding and then apply another pad and dressing over the top.

Collapsed Lung

If the patient has suffered an injury to the chest that has caused a puncture, this in turn creates an air leakage between the lung and the chest wall. The pleural space that resides here is usually full of negative pressure that allows the lung to compress and expand as we breathe. If you suspect this has occurred, use a stethoscope to listen to the breathing on both sides. One side will either feature diminished breathing sounds or no breathing at all.

This is likely to be accompanied by other symptoms, such as a difficulty in breathing and pain in the chest area. The skin may turn blue and the veins in the neck may be distended, while the windpipe often shifts away to the side of the good lung.

First, check for a chest wound and cover it immediately, as this could allow more air to enter the pleural space. Use a heavy dressing or tape to cover the wound. Air may accumulate in the pleural space under pressure, known as a pneumothorax, which will cause the patient's condition to worsen quickly and dramatically.

If this occurs, push your finger through the wound into the chest to encourage the air to escape. The air will hiss as it does so and the lung will expand partially. This may save your patient's life and will confirm your diagnosis of a collapsed lung.

If there is no chest wound, you will need to allow the air to escape another way. Push a needle through the wall of the chest on the top side of the second to fourth rub, in the line directly down from the armpit.

Seal the entry wound with a non-air permeable dressing and seal it only on three sides so that air can still escape, but cannot enter the wound.

Now, administer oxygen through a tank at five liters per minute. Keep a close eye on the breathing rate and quality and assist with breathing if it becomes necessary.

Anaphylactic Shock

For a patient who has had an allergic reaction to a food or an insect bite, the symptoms can appear very quickly and can worsen rapidly, becoming life threatening in a matter of minutes. Symptoms may include itching and a raised rash, swollen extremities, eyes and lips, a feeling of faintness, swelling in the mouth, wheezing, nausea and collapse.

First, ask the patient if they are carrying medication for the reaction – many people who have allergies severe enough to cause anaphylactic shock are aware of the condition and carry medication to treat it quickly, because there is often not enough time to call emergency services even in a normal situation.

Whether you can use the patient's medication or must administer your own, the treatment is an adrenaline injection. Make sure to have some in stock and read the instructions carefully – preferably you should already have familiarized yourself with the tool. Once you have performed the injection, hold the syringe in place for ten seconds. The symptoms should begin to dissipate very quickly, though the patient should then rest on their back with their legs raised to encourage blood flow.

Poison

Poison comes in many forms and is especially likely in a survival scenario, where people may be relying on unfamiliar substances for food and can choose the wrong plant for their dinner. Most poison victims will vomit as their body automatically attempts to reject the poison. They may also feel pain or a burning sensation and they may lose consciousness.

Contrary to what may seem common sense, do not try to induce vomiting, though you can encourage them to spit out anything left in the mouth. Nor should you give the person any food or water to ingest. Instead, ask what the person has swallowed or whether they have inhaled poisonous fumes and keep a close eye on them in case they fall unconscious. If this happens, always place them in the recovery position in case of vomit. If the poison is on their clothing or skin, clean the area with warm water.

A hospital or medical facility usually has antidotes on hand but, as this is likely not an option for you, your best bet is to use activated charcoal, which binds to the poison and prevents it from being absorbed into the patient's bloodstream.

Be aware that activated charcoal can cause dehydration, so, after following the instructions carefully and allowing it to take effect and the patient to recover, you should make sure to encourage consumption of plenty of water.

Burns and Scalds

If your patient has been burned from fire, a hot surface or a chemical, your first step will be to stop the burning from occurring. You may need to douse them with water, smother them with a blanket or remove the patient from the vicinity of the material causing the burn.

Next, remove any clothing or accessories that are close to the affected area of skin – unless it is stuck to that skin, because in this case you will cause additional damage. Cool the area with lukewarm running water for around 20 minutes, but keep the patient warm with blankets as you do so because there will always be a risk of hypothermia during this process. This cleaning process will also serve to wash out any chemicals or residue on the burn.

Once the affected area is cooled, cover it with plastic wrap. You should aim to use it as a layer rather than a wrap. Treat the pain with painkillers.

Electric Shock

Be very aware of your own safety if a patient is suffering or has suffered an electric shock. The source is unlikely to deactivate by itself, so you will want to immediately find the source of the current and switch it off. In a survival situation, this may be a generator; if the power is still running, it could be the mains to the building the patient is in.

The effects of the shock will depend on the voltage as well as how the current traveled through the patient's body and their overall levels of health. Do not move the patient, but do apply a blanket to keep them warm and cover any burns with a sterile dressing. Make sure that you check for breathing and circulation, as a severe electric shock can cause the heart to stop. Perform CPR as quickly as possible.

Heart Attack

Knowing the symptoms of a heart attack can save a patient's life. If a person complains that they are suffering from chest pain, ask them where specifically the pain is and what it feels like. The pain of a heart attack is usually located in the center of the chest or the left side and feels like squeezing or pressure.

The pain may also appear to be "traveling" around the body, usually down one arm or both arms or sometimes into the patient's jaw, abdomen area or back.

Sit the patient somewhere comfortable and give them an aspirin tablet of a 300 mg dosage. Ask if they have any history of heart problems and, if so, if they have the appropriate medicine with them or somewhere accessible. If the heart attack worsens, you may need to perform CPR to resolve a cardiac arrest.

Seizures

Your priority if a patient suffers from a seizure is to protect their ability to breathe – do your best to keep their airway clear if they vomit. Turn the patient onto their side and use a padded object as a bite block to prevent damage from involuntary biting actions.

Try to prevent the patient from injuring themselves by using any available padding, such as a sleeping bag or cushion. Loosen their clothing and restrain them if necessary, making sure to keep them on their side.

Most seizures stop within a couple of minutes, but the patient will suffer after effects including confusion and sometimes difficulty in breathing. As a second seizure may also sometimes follow, it's important to watch the patient closely for at least an hour or so after.

As and when the patient is able to communicate, ask whether they have a history of seizures and are taking any medication that should be administered. Ask if they are diabetic and, if so, give them a sugary drink or snack to regulate their blood sugar levels as an imbalance can sometimes be a cause of seizures.

Asthma Attack

Most asthma sufferers carry an inhaler but, in a survival situation, your patient may be stranded without one or may have run out of medication. Keep your patient calm, as panic exacerbates the problem dramatically.

Administer oxygen to the patient at ten liters per minute, followed by your bronchodilator. If your patient is still suffering a severe attack, administer an adrenaline shot (check first whether your patient suffers from heart problems such as angina and do not administer if this is the case).

Finally, give your patient a corticosteroid tablet to reduce the inflammation that the attack has caused in their airways. This should be done as soon as possible because it is a delayed action tablet and your patient will not feel the effects for several hours. Continue to administer this over the next few days, slowly reducing the dosage over time.

Blood Clot

A blood clot can form anywhere in the body and travel until it finally arrives in the lung and causes a pulmonary embolism, preventing the lung from transferring oxygen to the heart. Look for pain, warmth or swelling if a patient complains of discomfort and you suspect a blood clot may be likely, for example if the patient has been sitting still for a long time or is dehydrated or obese.

If your patient complains of chest pains, is coughing and may have blood present in the cough, feels light headed and is short of breath and has an irregular heartbeat, the clot may already have reached the lung.

Give your patient a 325 mg aspirin tablet to swallow and administer oxygen at 10 liters per minute. Dose them with a blood thinner and then a maintenance anticoagulant.

Hypothermia

Human beings shiver to generate heat in a situation where the temperature has dropped, but this can only help for so long and it can also only be maintained for so long. If your patient has stopped shivering, this means they are entering a state of hypothermia. It can occur through exposure to extremely cold weather or by exposure to cold water. In the latter case, the patient may also hyperventilate.

Assume that any patient you have found in a cold environment is suffering from hypothermia. Watch for confusion and an altered mental state and even delusions. Use a thermometer to check the patient's temperature to confirm your diagnosis.

At between 91.4 and 98.6 degrees Fahrenheit, the patient will be experiencing mild hypothermia. By the time it has dropped to 71.6 to 85.2 degrees, the hypothermia is severe. Without treatment, once the shivering has stopped, the body temperature will drop continually and quickly.

Remove any wet clothing and replace it with either dry clothing or blankets and sleeping bags. Cover the head and neck to insulate and, if possible, ask two warm people to sit on either side of the patient. The patient will not be able to increase the temperature of the interior of the sleeping bag or blankets for themselves (much as you warm the blankets around yourself when you go to bed each evening) so use hot water bottles (you can use a canteen warmed over a fire and wrapped in blankets), a second person inside the sleeping bag or under the blankets, a hairdryer or even wrapped warm rocks to do this for them.

DO NOT rub the skin or ask the patient to move around or immerse them in a warm bath. This can cause heart problems. You need to bring the body temperature up gently and gradually using the techniques described above. Administer sugary drinks once the patient has begun to recover to prevent a severe drop in blood sugar.

Frostbite

If frostbite has accompanied hypothermia, it will cause numbness and white skin with a yellow or blue tint. You will need to warm the area rapidly but do not do this unless you can maintain the warmer temperature once achieved – if it cools again, the damage will be even worse. Immerse the area in warm water at a temperature of around 98 to 104 degrees Fahrenheit and keep the water circulating using your hand. It's usually better to use a container in which the skin will not touch the sides.

Warming the skin can take up to 45 minutes and will be complete once the skin is again pliable and the color and feeling have both returned. If the frostbite has caused blisters, treat them with a sterile bandage and antiseptic ointment.

Heatstroke

The opposite problem to hypothermia, over exposure to heat can cause issues just as severe. The patient will appear to be confused and will feel dizzy and nauseous and may behave irrationally. The skin may actually feel cool to the touch but the core temperature has risen beyond manageable levels.

The patient may also develop a rash, vomiting, shock, seizures, weakness and unconsciousness if the problem reaches serious levels. Remove the patient from any obvious heat sources and remove their clothing. Drench them with crushed ice and water or place ice packs behind their neck, in the groin area and under the armpits. Alternatively, soak towels with ice water and cover the patient, changing them regularly to keep them cool. You can also immerse the patient in a cold body of water, keeping a close eye on their temperature to prevent it from dipping below 99.5 to 100 degrees Fahrenheit.

As the patient reaches this temperature, taper off whatever you are doing to cool them. Attend to their hydration by giving them water to sip constantly over the next couple of hours – and extra water over the next day to 36 hours.

Treatment for Wounds and Injuries

This category of medical need is likely to be present during a first aid situation, but it can also happen at any moment on any normal day. Whether your patient was cutting vegetables and accidentally sliced through their skin or was walking outside the shelter and developed a blister, your services will be required.

When evaluating a wound, start by asking the patient to explain what happened to them. Assume that the wound will need to be cleaned to prevent infection from setting in. Ask your patient if they are allergic to any medications you may need to use. Finally, ask the patient to show you their range of motion so that you can ascertain whether the injury has caused greater problems than are visible.

Severe Bleeding

A cut or laceration that penetrates the deep layers of the skin will lead to major bleeding. If this bleeding is dark in color and steady in seeping from the wound, it is from a vein. If it is bright red and spurting from the wound, it is arterial. Some injuries may have both.

Control the loss of blood using pressure directly over the wound. Your patient will begin to show serious effects after losing 1.5 pints of blood and will be in serious jeopardy if more than four pints are lost – you want to control the bleeding as quickly as possible to prevent this from happening.

Pressure will often be enough to stop the bleeding. If the wound is on an arm or leg, you can also use elevation above heart level to help stem it.

If pressure is not enough, you may need to put additional pressure on a nearby major artery at a location where it is close enough to the surface to be reached from the exterior.

For a scalp wound, apply pressure at the temples. For a neck wound, apply pressure at the jugular. For an arm wound, you will find the artery at the front of the armpit. Apply pressure on the inner thigh for a leg wound above the knee and the back of the knee for a wound below the knee. The very base of the ankle where it connects with the foot is the pressure point for a foot wound, the point where the pelvis meets the thigh for a thigh wound and the wrist for a hand wound.

If the wound continues to bleed, administer a tourniquet above the wound; in other words, applied tightly and securely between the wound and the heart, to limit the amount of blood that can flow towards it. Be extremely careful when using a tourniquet as the area of the body you are using it on does still need oxygen from the blood and leaving it in place for too long will cause limb loss and other serious issues. Loosen it every ten minutes at a minimum and remove it as soon as you are comfortable that the serious bleeding has been stemmed.

Release pressure and flush the wound with sterile water or an antiseptic solution. Flushing a wound involves making sure that a stream of fluid is flowing over the wound, washing any embedded dirt away from the body. The stream will need to be relatively forceful to make this happen, so it's best to give the wound at least an hour to clot over before doing this.

You'll want to use at least a pint of fluid per wound, which can be administered using a syringe. DO NOT soak the wound, as you will essentially be "stewing it in its own juices" as the bacteria washes into the water.

Pack it with bandages to keep pressure on the wound even once it is dressed and prevent the bleeding from starting again. Put the most pressure from your dressing on the place where the bleeding was occurring in the case of a large area wound.

Cover the bandages with a dry dressing and make sure to change both bandages and dressings at least twice a day while the wound is healing. If bleeding continues, you can use a hemostatic product to assist.

Removing Foreign Objects

During the first aid chapter of this book, we mentioned that you will sometimes come across injuries where a foreign object is embedded in a wound. At the site of the injury, it is never a good idea to remove these objects as you cannot know whether the object itself is preventing a more serious bleed.

Once your patient has been transferred to a safe location with plenty of medical supplies available, you can more safely investigate the foreign object and attempt to ascertain whether removing it will cause serious damage. If removing it does cause serious bleeding, follow the steps in the previous section.

If medical help will be available in the long term, such as if you are involved in a short term disaster emergency, NEVER remove the foreign object yourself – wait for a medical professional. If you must do so yourself, be aware that your actions can have serious repercussions and do your best to have the equipment and helping hands available to deal with them.

Closing Open Wounds

Deep wounds may have trouble closing by themselves. There are plenty of methods available to assist with closure. For instance, you can use a butterfly closure, which attaches on either side of the wound and connects over the top of it.

You may also use medical grade glue by holding the edges of the laceration together and running the glue along the wound. Keep the wound held in place until the glue dries, then simply leave it be – the glue will peel away by itself as the wound heals.

If all else fails, you can even use duct tape to close a wound – anything that will hold the edges together and relieve some of the pressure of the open wound from the patient's body. If you use tape, approximate the shape of a butterfly closure and make sure to place tape across the wound all along its length to keep it aligned.

Scalp wounds tend to bleed more freely than other areas of the body. To close a scalp wound, use medical glue along the laceration and then twirl the hair along each side of it into thick strands, which can be tied together across the wound using string to help keep its edges pressed together.

Be aware that there are some circumstances in which it is not a good idea to close a wound. Specifically, you should not do so until the injury has been thoroughly and properly cleaned, as doing so will trap bacteria and other dirty material inside the body, hugely increasing – if not guaranteeing – the chances of infection. Any bite from an animal should not be closed, nor any wound that has lingering bacteria or toxins in it. Keeping it open allows you to continue cleaning it over time, helping to prevent infection. Make sure to use antibacterial cleaning materials and antibiotic cream to help stave off infection.

Bandaging a Wound

This is a skill that takes practice, so set aside some time before any emergency occurs to try out your techniques. If you can attend a first aid class, this will be one of the skills you will be taught – doing so is to be highly recommended.

As a general rule, you will want to secure your bandages firmly but not too tightly, as this can cut off circulation. If the patient's skin or nails become discolored or they experience a tingling or numbness, the bandage is too tight. A second rule of thumb is to use a square knot when tying a bandage in place.

- Hand Bandage: Position the patient's hand so that it is sitting naturally, with the fingers and palm slightly curled. Use padding or gauze between the fingers and a wrap the bandage in a figure of eight around the palm.

- Wrist Bandage: Wrap the bandage around the wrist three times and then over the top of the hand. Finally, take it through the space between thumb and fingers and across the palm.

- Body Bandage: Begin bandaging from the front and side of the injury. Wrap using spiral turns.

- Joint Bandage: Begin as above, making diagonal turns above and below the joint in a figure of eight pattern. Ensure the joint is slightly bent so that it is sitting naturally.

- Shoulder Bandage: Lay a triangular bandage at a downward angle so that it is pointing across the chest. Tie the ends under the opposite armpit, then roll the end on the injured side a few turns and secure with a knot.

Burns

How severe a burn is depends on how much of the surface of the patient's skin it has affected and how deep the injury goes.

- First Degree: This can be as simple as a sunburn and will involve warm skin, a red appearance and pain. Use a cool, wet cloth to relieve the area and provide ibuprofen for the pain. Aloe vera gel is also very effective for relieving the pain.

- Second Degree: This level of burn will involve blisters with red rings around them. The wound will likely weep clear fluid and swell up. Remove any tight clothing or jewelry near the wound in case of swelling and run cool (NOT cold) water over it for 15 minutes. Provide ibuprofen for pain and anesthetic ointment for the wound itself. Do not lance the blisters unless they are large and cover the wound with a non-stick dressing.

- **Third Degree:** This severe type of burn is difficult to treat in the absence of true medical facilities. Watch for shock, particularly if the burn is large. The burn will be deep enough to penetrate the deepest layers of the skin and possibly the fat and muscle below and may appear charred in color, or white. Administer plenty of fluids and cool the burn with running water. Use silver sulfadiazine cream to prevent infection and cover with celox combat gauze to protect the area.

If you are unable to obtain the medical supplies described above, you can use vinegar to prevent infections by applying a compress soaked in a solution of half vinegar, half cool water. You can also use a pure witch hazel compress or soak the burn in a warm bath with a quarter cup of baking soda added to it. Even black tea bags can be helpful, as their tannic acid will help to draw the heat from the burn. Use two or three tea bags in cool water and apply it using a compress. Honey can also be used in place of the celox combat gauze as it will prevent bacteria from entering the wound; it should be covered with plastic wrap using tape to hold the wrap in place.

Animal or Human Bites

Feral or wild animals or even humans often use their teeth as a form of attack or defense. Your primary concern is to remove the bacteria from the wound, as these will be among the dirtiest injuries of all and are prime territory for severe infection.

Flush the wound and refrain from closing it. Instead, clean it frequently and apply antibiotic cream. If possible, also administer antibiotic tablets.

In the case of a snake bite, make sure to keep the victim as calm as possible to reduce the risk of increased blood flow carrying the venom through the circulatory system. Keep the victim still for the same reason. As the anti venom is unlikely to be available to you, clean the bite thoroughly to remove excess venom and position the limb below heart level to slow the venom from being transported. Wrap with bandages tightly and continue those bandages further up the limb than usual. The patient should be kept at rest with the bite lower than their heart for one to two days.

Soft Tissue Injuries

These injuries include cuts, abrasions, bruises, scratches and contusions – essentially, any injury that has damaged the surface of the skin but has not penetrated through to the deeper layers.

Wash the wound to ensure that it is clean from dirt and bacteria that may cause infection, use an antiseptic ointment to clear any infection already present and use ibuprofen to treat any pain. If you are unable to obtain ibuprofen or you have run out, you can instead use a natural version such as garlic or raw honey.

Blisters

Cover a blister that is just beginning to form with moleskin to prevent it from worsening. If you do not have any available, use a simple Band Aid. If the blister has already formed, resist the temptation to pop it if it is small.

If it is large, however, disinfect the area and sterilize the needle you intend to use before piercing the side of the blister to enable the fluid to drain out of it. Do not peel away the skin, but cover the blister with a dressing to protect it from infection and apply antibiotic cream. In the event that none is available, use a cold compress soaked in salt water or apply witch hazel three times a day.

Splinters

Wherever possible, splinters should be removed by cutting the skin until you are able to reach the end and pull the splinter out with tweezers. Make sure to disinfect the area before doing so and sterilize your tweezers and you may want to use antibiotics after the removal or if you see any swelling or redness.

Stings and Insect Bites

Whether or not you were successful in swatting the culprit after a patient has been stung, be aware that bees and wasps send out pheromone signals that let their comrades know an attack is happening, so you should always leave the area. If the sting is from a wasp, use tweezers to remove the stinger. Clean the area around the sting and place anesthetic cream over it and a cold pack to reduce the swelling and ease the pain. Use Benadryl to control the itching that stings so often cause and ibuprofen for any pain.

Watch your patient carefully in the minutes after the sting, as some will have an allergic reaction and will appear faint, short of breath, dizzy and itchy. Some will experience extreme swelling around the area of the bite. As with any other allergic reaction, this will require the application of an adrenaline injection quickly to prevent the allergic reaction from closing off the person's airway.

Rarely, you will come across a dangerous spider bite from a species such as the black widow or the brown recluse.

- Black Widow: The area will be red and also raised and you may be able to see two puncture marks. The patient will report severe pain and may soon begin to experience cramping, pain in the abdomen, nausea, faintness, chest pain, shortness of breath, weakness and disorientation. The combination of symptoms will likely differ for each patient.

- Brown Recluse: These bites tend to be painless just after they occur, but after a while begin to itch and feel painful and the patient will also begin to display a fever, nausea and blisters near the bite.

What's actually happening as these symptoms appear is that the body, having activated its immune response to deal with the venom, has no real idea what to do about it and will begin to damage itself as a response, killing off blood cells and stopping clots from forming.

Wash the area of the bite and apply ice to swelling and pain. Administer pain medication and ask the patient to rest in bed. If the patient is experiencing muscle cramps, give them a warm bath – but only if you are sure that the bite was NOT from a brown recluse, as heat should never be applied to this kind of bite. Give antibiotics if available to prevent infection.

A scorpion sting can be lethal in some parts of the world. Be aware that scorpions are usually active in the night time. Watch for symptoms including pain or tingling or even numbness around the sting as well as sweating, weakness, extra saliva in the mouth, a restless and irritable demeanor, a difficulty in swallowing and rapid breathing and heart rate.

Wash the area and remove any tight clothing and jewelry from around it. Apply a cold compress and give the patient Benadryl. Make sure the patient remains calm to ensure that the poison spreads more slowly and keep food to a minimum if their throat has swollen. Administer pain relievers.

Treating Fractures and Dislocations

Damage to a patient's skeleton comes in two forms: open or closed. The former involves a broken or dislocated bone with pierced skin either from the bone itself or another trauma. The latter involves no damage to the skin itself, with the break or dislocation entirely under the surface.

Open fractures are much more dangerous to your patient as an open wound is obviously more susceptible to blood loss and also infection. When the wound is serious enough to have affected the bone, those infections can travel deeper into the body faster and can threaten the patient's life.

Your first task will be to properly evaluate the situation, as always. Remove clothing from around the break using scissors and look for any bleeding or signs of an open wound. Look around the injury for any changes in the patient's coloration, such as if the skin is pale or has turned blue. Check the patient's pulse to be sure that it is strong and steady.

Closed Breaks

In the case of a closed fracture, look at the shape of the limb that has broken. Is it still sitting in the same configuration you would expect if it was not broken?

If so, the break has not deformed the limb and you will simply need to apply a splint to keep it from moving and allow the bone to begin to heal.

If, however, the bone is not lying at the correct angle or the two halves of the break are now separated by a space, you will need to attempt to reposition the bone. Be aware that this will cause intense pain for the patient so you may want to enlist help to keep them still and you should ALWAYS provide full information about your intentions before you begin.

To reposition the displaced bone, apply a pulling force that increases steadily along the normal axis of that limb's alignment. At the same time, apply counter traction on the opposite side of the injury. If you meet with resistance, you may need to rock the limb very gently or even accentuate the deformity so that the bone can clear anything that is obstructing its path and return to its usual position. DO NOT ever attempt to reposition a spine injury.

Splinting a break involves immobilizing it using the strong area above and below the broken bone for support. You can use anything sturdy that you have to hand, from a stick or pole to a pad or piece of cardboard. Place the solid object alongside the break and use bandages, tape or any other tying mechanism to make firm ties at regular intervals all along it, taking care to avoid the site of the break itself.

You should do this with the body part at a natural angle that reflects that limb in motion. In other words, a hand should be gently clutching and an elbow or knee should be gently bent. Try to elevate the injured area to keep the swelling down.

Once the splint has been applied, regularly check the circulation by looking for discolored skin or pinching nails. Swelling during the healing process can sometimes cause the splint to cut off circulation and will require you to loosen the fastenings.

However, there are a few circumstances in which a simple splint will not work:

- Broken Jaw: To immobilize a broken jaw, tie a bandage across the chin and backwards horizontally behind the base of the skull. Tie a second bandage under the jaw and upwards to the top of the head. Be aware that this injury can cause nausea, so make sure your knots can be undone at speed.

- Breaks Around the Hand: Place a bandage on a flat surface and a rolled bandage on top of it. Ask the patient to place their hand over the top of the rolled bandage so it is in a position of gently gripping. Wrap the bandage over the hand, padding between the fingers but making sure to leave the tips of the fingers clear so that you can check for circulation.

- **Finger Breaks:** Use the next finger along as the splint, placing padding between them and taping above and below the break.

- **Slings:** For any injury to the hand, fingers, wrist or arm, you can create a sling to support the area while it heals. Place one corner of a triangular bandage in behind the neck and bring the rest down across the chest and under the arm. Bring the bandage back up to the neck from in front of the arm and secure behind the neck. You can use a bandage tied across the chest and under the opposite armpit to keep the arm from swinging if necessary. If you do not have a bandage available, you can also use sturdy pins to attach the arm of the person's clothing to the chest of that item of clothing.

- **Rib Fractures:** The action of breathing can be very painful for a patient who has broken a rib, but taping the area by firmly wrapping a bandage around the chest can provide some comfort. If the rib is fractured, follow the procedure to identify and treat a punctured lung before taping.

Open Breaks

In the case of an open break, first make sure to stop any bleeding using the techniques discussed earlier in this book. Be aware that applying pressure will cause extreme discomfort to the patient so be as gentle as you are able while still being effective.

Next, immobilize the area and apply ice packs to relieve the swelling. Watch for signs of shock and follow the procedure to clean and dress the wound outlined earlier, to ensure that infection does not set in. Once you have addressed the open wound, you can follow the same procedures as a closed wound to splint the break.

Dislocations

If a bone has been pulled from its joint, it will be very clear that something is amiss. The joint will hang or sit strangely and appear deformed and motion in that area will be severely limited. In some cases, the problem will solve itself spontaneously, but not always.

You will want to attempt to correct the dislocation as quickly as possible, once you have completed your full evaluation of the patient. As time goes on, swelling in the area will make the process both more difficult and more painful for the patient. Be aware, also, that this is going to be an incredibly painful process for the patient, so you may need a second set of hands to help restrain them as you work.

With the joint held stable (this is another area in which a second person can be very helpful), use a firm and slow pulling action to pull the bone away from the joint to allow it to realign itself. Now push the bone back in line with the joint socket and allow it to revert to its usual position. The body wants to do this, so you should meet with little resistance.

Once you have realigned the dislocation, splint or bandage as you would after a fracture. Just like a bone break, it can take significant time for the area to heal.

Treating Infectious Diseases

In the aftermath of a disaster, the likelihood of infectious diseases is heightened. Finding yourself stranded in unknown environments can also be problematic – as, of course, can changes in your own environment or even the release of a biological weapon. Some infectious diseases are of the kind that we deal with every day, such as the flu; others are much rarer.

Though you may be lucky enough to be sheltering in an environment free of some of the planet's nastiest diseases, it is always best to be prepared to face any or all of them. After all, there is no way to predict changes in the planetary environment after a disaster and you may also be faced by a situation in which a member of your party contracted a disease during travels prior to the disaster. And while it's impossible to cover every single potential disease in the span of one book, we will look at the most likely culprits if your patient begins showing signs of distress.

Treating some of these diseases may be difficult without the aid of a doctor for diagnosis and a medical facility for support and medication. However, you can still provide aid if you are able to scavenge for medical supplies in the surrounding area. Be very, very careful indeed when administering medications if you are not completely sure what the symptoms a patient is showing really mean. As you are not a medical professional, a firm diagnosis may not be within your power. Make sure you have gathered a full history of that patient's travel and are aware of the likelihood of their coming into contact with a particular disease before taking further steps and only ever move ahead with treatment if you are certain.

Influenza

More commonly known as "the flu", this disease comes in many forms and is highly infectious. If a member of your party contracts it, keep them as isolated as possible and pay attention to hygiene, as flu can be spread through breath, touch and bodily fluids. Make sure to wear gloves and a face mask when administering to a patient to prevent spreading the disease to yourself and then on to others.

Symptoms will include coughs, fevers, sore throat, a blocked nose, bodily aches, headaches and fatigue. Vomiting and diarrhea are sometimes also present, though not always.

Most patients will recover within a couple of weeks if they are encouraged to get plenty of bed rest and you make sure to administer fluids and fever medication such as ibuprofen. The danger of flu is much higher, however, in the elderly and small children and also pregnant women, so pay extra attention to these patients while they are showing symptoms.

Lyme Disease

This illness is surprisingly common in the United States, especially in the summer and first part of the fall, and is also known to occur in Europe, Australia, China and Japan. It is carried by ticks and the first symptom is usually a skin lesion that appears at the site of the tick bite around three days to one month after it occurs.

The lesion will appear to be a red spot that expands into a circle or oval that has irregular edges surrounding slightly paler skin. It will feel warm and may itch or feel as though it is burning.

The patient will also experience symptoms similar to the flu, including aches in the muscles, a low fever, joint pain, nausea and loss of appetite, coughing and a sore throat, swollen lymph glands, pain in the abdomen, sore or swollen eyes and an aversion to light. All but the tiredness and aches will disappear within three weeks.

This disease must be treated with antibiotics as, if it is left untreated, it can progress and cause damage to the nervous system and heart, as well as paralysis of the face. Use 100 mg of doxycycline given to the patient twice a day or 500 mg of amoxicillin administered three times daily for up to three weeks. For children, administer the latter medicine at a rate of 17 mg per kg of weight.

Meningitis

Easily spread among humans, this illness affects the respiratory system and usually appears as a fever and headache with a stiff neck. The patient may have a skin rash and may be averse to light.

Meningitis is a serious disease that can easily worsen. If the rash begins to spread and coalesce into large areas of discoloration, the disease is becoming worse and life threatening symptoms, such as shock and failure of the respiratory system, may follow.

You will need to administer high doses of antibiotics. If you are unable to administer ceftriaxone intravenously, give the patient penicillin, cefixime, amoxicillin or trimethoprim. You may also give ciprofloxacin to party members who have been in contact with the victim.

Malaria

Caused by a bite from an infected mosquito, this disease is most prevalent in southeast Asia, South America, Oceania, the Middle East and sub-Saharan Africa. Incubation takes from eight to 40 days and symptoms may not appear for up to two months.

Symptoms of the disease appear much like a flu, including some combination of headache, sweating, tiredness, loss of appetite, aching, nausea, back ache and pale skin. Patients may suffer from diarrhea or vomiting.

The next stage of symptoms will include more intense fever and chills with sweating and headache and the potential for anemia or jaundice. These symptoms will appear in stages of one to eight hours and will then disappear for two or three days before beginning again. The fever symptom may be delayed.

Under normal circumstances, malaria would be diagnosed by looking for parasites in the blood under a microscope. However, as this will likely not be possible and there is no vaccine for malaria, the best treatment is prevention. If you are in an area where malaria is prevalent, make sure to wear clothing that covers the body during the feeding times of evening and night and use insect repellent.

Travelers to these areas also generally take a preventative regime of mefloquine at 250 mg per week. This should be begun up to two weeks before travel and then for a month after returning. It is not appropriate for pregnant women or those with a history of seizures or depression. For children, the dose is considerably lower; 63 mg for a child weighing 15 to 19 kg or 125 mg for weight of 20 to 30 kg or 188 mg for children weighing 31 to 45 kg.

Alternative medications include doxycycline, also not appropriate for pregnant women or children under the age of eight (with dosage for children over this age at 2 mg per kg of body weight), quinine, quinidine and chloroquine phosphate.

Eastern Equine Encephalitis
Mostly confined to the mid-Atlantic and the New England states in America, this disease is also found in Latin America and is also carried by mosquitoes. The illness takes up to ten days to incubate, though it may appear as quickly as four days after the bite.

At first, the sufferer will show many of the symptoms of flu, such as chills, fever, aches and pains and tiredness. These will last for up to two weeks. The later symptoms of this disease include headaches and an altered mental state, as well as weak breath and pale or even blue skin and seizures. The sufferer is also likely to suffer from periods of unconsciousness that eventually lead to a coma. The death rate from this disease is around one third and those who survive often suffer permanent mental consequences.

Watch for this disease particularly in the summer and early fall. Keep an eye on horses in the area, in which species it is likely to appear first. Unfortunately, there is neither a vaccine nor a cure for this disease, so you will only be able to keep the patient hydrated, warm and rested while their symptoms persist.

Trichinosis

This disease is spread through a larvae embedded in meat that is then consumed by humans. If you find yourself eating wild meat, make sure that it is most commonly spread because the meat has not been cooked properly – always be sure to prepare your food thoroughly.

If your patient shows signs of nausea, vomiting and diarrhea that continues longer than a couple of days, this disease may be the cause. It can go on for up to six weeks and, in the second week, leads to swelling, fever and aching, as well as weakness and rashes.

The larvae will die and calcify between six and 18 months after the person became infected. The treatment for this disease is not 100 percent effective and involves administering mebendazole.

West Nile Disease

Another disease spread by mosquitoes, this one appears all across the United States and the Middle East and West Asia, and is also carried by birds and small mammals. It is difficult to spread between humans, although it has been known to spread via organ transplant, blood transfusion or breast milk.

This disease most often appears in summer and autumn and has an incubation period of three to 14 days. At first, the patient will show symptoms akin to the common flu, with swollen lymph glands and loss of appetite. Watch for a rash on the body and an aversion to light. Be aware that some patients may experience convulsions and these should be watched for.

It's rare for a patient to die from West Nile Disease and many people experience no symptoms at all.

Keep the patient on bed rest and make sure they are hydrated and kept at a comfortable temperature. Make sure to reassure them, as some of the symptoms may include disorientation and loss of vision, or even paralysis, and these can be frightening to experience.

If you are aware that West Nile Disease is or has been a problem in your region in the past, be sure there is no standing water around your shelter to attract mosquitoes and limit your time spent outside in the dawn and dusk hours. Use insect repellant whenever possible when performing outdoor activity or traveling.

Rocky Mountain Spotted Fever

This disease is carried by parasites on ticks and appears mostly in the late spring and early summer in the southeastern portion of the United States. The average incubation period is one week, though it may vary from a couple of days to two weeks.

When the symptoms appear, they will be heralded by a sudden high fever. This will often be accompanied by a red and spotted rash that will often occur on the patient's ankles or wrists and then begin to spread. When it appears, the rash will lose its color when pressed. Later, the rash will darken and turn into blotches.

These symptoms may also be accompanied by headaches, aches, coughing, swelling in the hands, feet, eyelids and face and red eyes, as well as nausea and pain in the abdomen. The best treatment is 100 mg twice daily of doxycycline or 500 mg of tetracycline four times a day. These doses will be lower for children and the appropriate amount should be marked on the packaging.

Typhoid

This bacteria caused disease most often appears in places of bad hygiene and can be ingested in food or water. In a disaster scenario, it is more likely than usual to affect survivors.

It takes ten days to two weeks for symptoms to appear, after which the patient will display a fever and may experience pain in the abdomen and diarrhea. These may be accompanied by headaches and tiredness and a loss of appetite, as well as "rose spots" on the main portion of their body that lose their color if pressed.

The disease generally cures itself after three weeks to a month if the patient is kept hydrated and warm. Some cases are fatal or cause long term issues, however. If you are able to administer antibiotics, use ciprofloxacin or azithromycin at a dosage of 10 mg for every kg of body weight, twice a day for one week.

Hemorrhagic Fever

The most famous of these diseases is Ebola, but there are several versions in existence. They can all be spread easily between humans in bodily fluids of all kinds, so it's imperative that you protect yourself when treating a patient. Do not assume that these illnesses, including Lassa, Crimean-Congo and Marburg, are limited to certain countries. In a post disaster world, they could easily be carried with migrant survivors.

Between two and 21 days after exposure to Ebola, the patient will display a fever as well as a strong headache and pain in the abdomen. They may have a sore throat and vomiting or diarrhea a well as muscle pains and general weakness. As the disease worsens, so too will the vomiting and diarrhea and eventually the patient may collapse.

No direct treatment is available, so the best course of action is to administer to the symptoms as you are able. It is crucial to ensure the patient remains hydrated as the symptoms will cause a loss of fluids to dangerous levels.

Colorado Tick Fever

Another virus that is spread through ticks, this disease appears between early spring and late fall and is most prevalent in summer. It takes between three and six days to incubate and is also typified by a sudden fever, as well as a severe headache and other aches across the body. The patient may be averse to light and experience pain in the eyes and abdomen, as well as nausea.

Around 50 percent of patients will show a pattern to their fever. It will last for around three days, disappear for one to two days and then come back for another two to three days. It can take up to three weeks for the illness to resolve but some symptoms, such as tiredness and a feeling of weakness, may persist. Again, concentrate on administering to the symptoms of the disease and keeping the patient comfortable, rested and hydrated.

Leptospirosis

The organisms that cause this disease are passed on through animal urine and most commonly picked up by humans through contact with water or soil. They enter through open wounds in the skin and also through the eye or mouth.

The incubation period lasts for between two days and three weeks and the symptoms include fever and chills, nausea and vomiting, aches and headaches, swelling in the lymph glands and red eyes. After about a week, the patient will seem better for a few days, but then new symptoms will appear, including aches, nausea, vomiting, a skin rash of red or purple patches, a sore throat and enlarged organs.

Administer antibiotics: doxycycline twice a day at a dosage of 100 mg or tetracycline four times a day at 500 mg. Continue this for seven days.

Tularemia

Common across the world, this disease is spread either through the bite of a tick or by consuming a rabbit that has been infected. It takes three to six days to incubate but sometimes up to three weeks. The symptoms are numerous and appear in various combinations depending on the patient.

If the patient handled the rabbit, they may develop ulcers on their hands and swollen lymph glands in the elbow and armpit. Other symptoms include a sore throat, fever, headache, weight loss, conjunctivitis, chills and fever. The treatment for this illness in an emergency situation is doxycycline twice a day at 100 mg or tetracycline four times a day at 500 mg. An alternative is ciprofloxacin at 750 mg twice a day. Continue medication for up to three weeks.

Treating Chronic, Minor and Non-Infectious Illnesses

Some members of your party may arrive at your post disaster shelter with pre existing conditions. Others may develop disorders or catch minor illnesses as time goes on; such is the nature of life. Many of these issues are mild and represent more of a hindrance than a threat to life, but some are more serious.

While many of these illnesses will not do well without proper medical care, particularly in the long term, you can still improve the patient's quality of life and expand their chances of survival by administering the best aid possible under the circumstances.

Diabetes

A diabetes sufferer is unable to produce insulin to properly manage their sugar intake, which in turn can lead to high levels of sugar in the blood. This, over time, can cause a myriad of issues across the body as the organs deteriorate, so the most obvious and crucial treatment is to monitor their blood sugar levels and change the diet to reduce the amount of sugar included. This can be tough in a survival situation as most survival foods are deliberately packed with carbs to provide the most amount of calorie intake in the smallest package.

Two types of diabetes exist. The one in which injections of insulin are needed most often appears at a young age so your patient may already be aware of it. You will need a hefty amount of insulin stored at your shelter for this person and may need to scavenge for more at a local medical facility.

The other type typically appears later in life and requires more attention to dietary changes. However, in both cases, you must keep an eye on the patient at all times for high or low blood sugar levels, which can lead to emergency situations.

Low blood sugar manifests in weakness and sweating, as well as pain in the abdomen and hunger. The patient will likely exhibit strange behavior and feel confused. You need to give them sugar as quickly as possible. If they fall unconscious, place granules of sugar under the tongue to dissolve in the saliva. The total amount of carb they will need is 20 g.

The opposite but associated emergency is high blood sugar, which also causes confusion as well as shallow breathing, a breath odor that smells like fruit or nail polish remover, vomiting and intense thirst. The pulse will quicken and feel weak and the skin will appear dry. The patient must be given intravenous fluids and an insulin injection. However, before injecting them, you must measure the blood sugar level and adjust the dose accordingly.

Headaches and Migraines

Headaches are a common problem and can be caused by all sorts of issues. Unless it is associated with a head injury or comes accompanied by other serious symptoms, you can assume it is not life threatening (though you will always want to keep an eye on the patient in case more symptoms develop and keep in mind that a prolonged headache may be a symptom of a much more serious issue).

If the pain is in the temples and eyes and at the back of the neck, ask the patient to rest and give pain medication. A massage at the back of the neck can provide relief. If the headache is a migraine or cluster headache (the latter of which usually only manifests on one side of the head), there are no remedies but you can make the patient more comfortable with rest, a darkened room and oxygen.

A sinus headache appears around the sinuses and is often accompanied by throbbing, fever and nasal discharge. Give the patient an oral decongestant and an antibiotic if those other symptoms appear.

Commonly, headaches are caused by dehydration so ask the patient to drink water to relieve the symptoms.

Altitude Sickness

For this disorder, associated with low oxygen levels, prevention is better than cure. If you must ascend more than 3000 m for any reason, this should be done in several stages to give the body time to acclimatize as you go. Never sleep higher than 300 m above the place you slept the night before and, if you head above 3048 m, stop for up to four days for acclimatization and rest often while you are at that altitude. Use acetazolamide to stimulate the breath and help the body adjust.

High Blood Pressure

Many patients already suffering from this issue will have medication available, though you may need to scavenge to keep your supplies healthy. Monitor the blood pressure throughout the day using a blood pressure cuff as it will vary and watch for anything over 160/100, which can indicate complications.

If your patient experiences headaches along with blurred vision and nausea, they may be suffering from persistent hypertension. Keep them on bed rest and restrict salt from the diet. Avoid alcohol, caffeine and nicotine. Seek high blood pressure medications and continue to administer until the readings go back to normal.

Thyroid Disease

A lump on the thyroid just in front of and below the Adam's apple indicates issues with this organ, which is responsible for the hormones that regulate your metabolism. Usually this indicates a lack of iodine in the body so administer potassium iodide tablets (unless the patient is allergic to seafood).

If hyperthyroidism develops and the thyroid is over-producing, you will see symptoms including insomnia, tremors in the hand, nervousness, bulging eyes, sweating, weight loss, frequent defecations, weight loss and muscle weakness. Administer propylthiouracil or methimazole to block the function of the thyroid – if you know a member of your party suffers thyroid problems, consider stockpiling these ahead of time.

If hypothyroidism occurs, the opposite is happening: the thyroid is not producing enough hormone. The patient will be fatigued, constipated, have a poor appetite but weight gain, hair loss, signs of depression and an intolerance to cold. Look for thyroid medications such as synthroid and levothroid.

Heart Disease

If a patient is suffering heart problems, keep a close eye for the symptoms of a heart attack. These will include pain in the left arm and jaw and a crushing sensation in the chest, as well as sweating and weakness and pale skin. Give the patient aspirin to thin the blood and prevent clots and sit the patient at a 45 degree angle. Impose complete rest after the event and keep the patient calm to reduce the risk of an anxiety event straining the heart.

To prevent heart problems from reaching this stage, give the patient a small dosage of aspirin daily. One baby aspirin is usually sufficient.

Kidney Stones

The signs of a kidney stone include pain on one side of the patient's back that comes and goes and also travels as the stone itself moves across the body. The urine may be bloody and the patient may be feverish or chilled and nauseated. Kidney stones are known to occur repeatedly once they have happened to a patient once so, if a member of your party has had one in the past, pay close attention to them.

You should also make sure that patient stays hydrated, as dehydration is one of the main triggers. Decrease the amount of dairy and calcium rich foods in their diet (though not by too much, as they still need calcium).

When a kidney stone occurs, your priority is to help it move as quickly as possible through the patient's system so they can expel it. Ask the patient to drink eight or more glasses of water a day, or cranberry juice if available. Pain relief including ibuprofen can be administered when it is time to pass the stone through the urine.

Urinary Tract and Kidney Infections

If a urinary tract infection is left untreated, it can travel to the kidneys. The symptoms of a UTI include frequent need to use the bathroom and pain or burning when doing so, as well as difficulty passing urine despite the need to go.

If this is accompanied by pain on one side of the back, a fever and chills, bloody or cloudy urine, sweating and dysuria, the infection has spread and the patient will need antibiotics. Look for sulfamethoxazole, ampicillin or ciprofloxacin. When a UTI first presents, administer plenty of fluids, including cranberry juice if available, and warmth to the bladder region.

Fungal Infections

A fungal infection on any part of the body can be painful and is also contagious. Look for flaking, itching, burning, discolored nails and red skin.

Apply topical antifungal ointments to the area and wash it regularly. Keep it dry and make sure clothing and bedding is cleaned daily.

Tetanus

Spread through rust, splinters, insect bites, soil and feces, this infection is caused by the spores of bacteria and usually only occurs when the patient's skin is broken. Whenever a patient experiences any wound that breaks the skin, watch for sore muscles, irritability, weakness, lockjaw and problems swallowing. This will be followed by spasms that get worse over time, involuntary arching of the back, high blood pressure, fever, problems breathing and an irregular heart beat.

Administer antibiotics as quickly as possible to kill off the bacteria. Metronidazole at 500 mg twice daily or doxycycline at 100 mg twice daily will work. Keep the patient hydrated and wash the wound itself thoroughly and frequently, flushing it out with water to begin with.

Eczema, Hives and Hay Fever

Two allergies that are very common in the modern world are eczema on the skin, which manifests as red and patchy areas of skin and itchy or flaky areas, and hay fever, which manifests similarly to a cold or flu. In the former case, apply a steroid cream such as hydrocortisone or clobetasol (the latter is stronger and for worse cases) according to the instructions on the packaging. In the latter case, give the patient antihistamines daily.

Hives generally appear if the patient has been exposed to something they are allergic to or in the presence of cold or heat after exposure to extreme temperatures. Watch for swelling, red welts with irregular borders and thickened patches of skin, as well as itching or fever. Administer an antihistamine until the symptoms subside.

Poison Ivy

If a patient has been exposed to this toxic plant (which you should learn to recognize and avoid by its distinctive three leaf structure), it will cause a red and itchy rash. Make sure to launder any clothing, as the oil that causes the reaction can stay active for a very long time, using a detergent that removes oil and resin.

The rash will eventually disappear but, to treat the painful symptoms, administer Benadryl four times a day in 25 to 50 mg doses.

Diarrhea

Many illnesses cause diarrhea, but it can also appear on its own if the patient has eaten or drunk contaminated items. It will cause severe dehydration so you will need to keep your patient drinking plenty of water, but they should avoid eating solid food for at least 12 hours. Once the diarrhea has ceased, give the patient oral rehydration salts to rebalance their hydration levels. If you do not have any available, mix 6 tsps of sugar with one of salt and half of potassium chloride, as well as a pinch of baking soda, and mix with plenty of water. As you care for the patient, keep a close eye for other symptoms that may indicate the diarrhea is a symptom rather than an isolated problem.

Shingles

This skin eruption occurs in patients who have experienced chicken pox; the virus remains behind in the body and manifests again as a rash that looks like crops of blisters. The patient may also experience a headache, feel tired and be sensitive to light. Keep the rash clean and covered with a light dressing. The problem will resolve itself within a month but, if the victim's condition worsens or the rash has appeared on the mouth, eyes or genitals, you can consider giving them acyclovir five times a day in 800 mg doses.

Conclusion

This book cannot make you a doctor – only years of training at a medical school would be able to do that. In the event of a serious disaster, you cannot replace a trained medical professional and there are some maladies you will not be able to help with at all. You cannot, for example, perform surgery.

But that doesn't mean that the skills you have learned over the course of these pages cannot save a life. Indeed, with the knowledge you have gained, you now have the potential to save many lives.

You will be able to give your loved ones the best chance of survival and full health after a disaster, whether or not help is on the way. You will be able to administer first aid efficiently and quickly and care for your patient until they have recovered. You know how to diagnose some of the most likely issues you and your family will encounter and you know how best to tackle them.

We all hope that disaster never strikes. If we are lucky, it never will. But if the worst does come to pass, you have now become worth your weight in gold to the people who will be relying on you for medical care.

Special Thanks

I would like to give special thanks to all the readers from around the globe who chose to share their kind and encouraging words with me.

Knowing even just one person found this book helpful means the world to me.

If you've benefited from this book at all, I would be honored to have you share your thoughts on it, so that others would get something valuable out of this book too.

Your reviews are the fuel for my writing soul, and I'd be **<u>forever grateful</u>** to see *your* review, too.

Thank you all!